OSTEOPOROSIS

EVERYTHING ABOUT HEALING

OSTEOPOROSIS

DR. A. RAMOS

Contents

INTRODUCTION

A medical disorder called osteoporosis is characterized by the weakening of bones, which increases the risk of fractures and increases bone fragility. Since the term "osteoporosis" literally translates to "porous bones," it emphasizes the loss of mass and density in the bones. Because this illness frequently shows no symptoms until a fracture happens, early detection and prevention are essential.

Reduced bone density and quality, known as osteoporosis, increases the risk of fractures, especially in the hip, spine, and wrist. Although osteoporosis causes an acceleration of the natural aging process, which leads to brittle and porous bones, bone density loss is a normal aspect of aging.

Age, gender (more prevalent in women, particularly after menopause), family history, hormonal fluctuations, insufficient calcium and vitamin D intake, sedentary lifestyle, smoking, excessive alcohol intake, and specific medical conditions or drugs are risk factors for osteoporosis.

Osteoporosis can be prevented and managed with a change in lifestyle, sufficient calcium and vitamin D intake, weight-bearing activity, and, in certain situations, medication. By enabling prompt intervention through bone density testing, early detection lowers the risk of osteoporosis-related fractures. Maintaining bone health and stopping the progression of osteoporosis require an understanding of and attention to risk factors.

CHAPTER ONE

What Osteoporosis Means

A medical disorder called osteoporosis is characterized by the weakening of bones, which raises the risk of fractures and results in a decrease in bone density. Because osteoporosis patients lose both bone mass and bone mineral density, their bones become porous and brittle. This increases the risk of fractures, especially in weight-bearing bones like the wrists, hips, and spine.

Principal Aspects of Osteoporosis:

Bone Density Reduction: The measurement of minerals (including calcium) in bone tissue, bone mineral density (BMD) is correlated with osteoporosis. The bones became weaker as a result of this density loss.

Microarchitectural Alterations: The typical architecture of bones is disrupted, among other modifications to the interior structure of bones. This adds to the heightened brittleness of bones.

Increased Fracture Risk: One of the main symptoms of osteoporosis is an increased risk of fractures, particularly in the wrist, hip, and vertebrae (spine). Normal activity or mild trauma can cause these fractures.

Asymptomatic Nature: Until a fracture happens, osteoporosis frequently shows no symptoms. Because people might not become aware of the illness until they feel discomfort or fractures, early detection and preventive measures are crucial.

Women who have gone through menopause are more likely to develop osteoporosis because of hormonal changes, namely a drop in estrogen levels. Nonetheless, it can impact both genders and all age groups. Osteoporosis can occur as a result of a number of risk factors, such as age, family history, low calcium and vitamin D consumption, sedentary lifestyle, and specific medical conditions or drugs.

Bone density testing, such as dual-energy X-ray absorptiometry (DXA) scans, which measure bone mineral density at various places in the body, is commonly used to make the diagnosis.

Osteoporosis can be managed and prevented by weight-bearing exercises, proper calcium and vitamin D intake, lifestyle changes, and, in certain situations, medicines. Reducing the risk of fractures, strengthening bones, and slowing down bone loss are the objectives. To manage osteoporosis and promote bone health, a multidisciplinary approach, thorough risk assessment, and early detection are crucial.

Reasons and Danger Elements

A complex illness, osteoporosis is caused by a confluence of environmental, hormonal, genetic, and lifestyle variables. It is essential to comprehend the causes and risk factors in order to identify high-risk individuals and put preventive measures in place. The main reasons and risk factors for osteoporosis are as follows:

1. Growing Older:

The main risk factor for osteoporosis is getting older. As we age, our bone density gradually declines and our risk of fractures rises.

2. Gender

Osteoporosis is more common in women, particularly after menopause. Accelerated bone loss is a result of the menopause-induced drop in estrogen levels.

3. Changes in Hormones:

An increased risk of osteoporosis can result from hormonal abnormalities, such as low testosterone in males or low estrogen in women, which can cause bone loss.

4. Family Background:

A hereditary propensity to osteoporosis or fractures may be indicated by a family history of the disorder. Bone structure and density can be influenced by genetic factors.

5. inadequate intake of calcium and vitamin D

Low calcium and vitamin D intake, which are vital for strong bones, can lead to a decrease in bone mass and a higher chance of fracture.

6. Low Mass:

Reduced bone mass and an elevated risk of osteoporosis may be linked to low body weight or a history of eating disorders.

7. A Sedentary Way of Life

Insufficient physical activity and weight-bearing exercises may be a factor in bone loss. Exercises involving weight bearing promote the growth of new bone and support bone density.

8. Smoking:

Because smoking may interfere with bone remodeling and lower bone density, it is considered a risk factor for osteoporosis.

9. Consumption of Alcohol Too Much:

Increased and prolonged alcohol use can have a detrimental effect on bone health and reduce bone density.

10. Health Issues:

Osteoporosis can be made more likely by a number of illnesses, including inflammatory bowel disease, celiac disease, rheumatoid arthritis, and hormone imbalances.

11. Drugs:

Long-term use of several drugs, such as anticonvulsants, glucocorticoids (steroids), and some cancer treatments, may exacerbate bone loss.

12. Past Breaks:

Those who have previously broken bones may be more susceptible to osteoporosis, particularly if the breaks were caused by little stress.

13. ethnicity

In comparison to other ethnic groups, populations that identify as Caucasian and Asian are typically more susceptible to osteoporosis.

14. Menopause:

Osteoporosis risk increases and bone loss is hastened in postmenopausal women due to a marked decrease in estrogen levels.

Together with bone density testing, a thorough evaluation of these risk factors aids medical practitioners in identifying patients who are more susceptible to osteoporosis. To lessen the effects of osteoporosis and improve bone health, preventive measures, dietary changes, and, where required, pharmaceutical interventions can be used. For early detection and prompt action, routine examinations and bone density testing are critical.

Signs and Quiet Character

Osteoporosis is commonly known as a "silent disease" since it usually worsens without causing any symptoms until a fracture. In the early stages of the disorder, there may be no symptoms, thus people may not become aware of their bone loss until they experience a fracture or other bone-related issue. The following are some important details about osteoporosis's symptoms and quiet nature:

1. Early Asymptomatic Stages:

Usually, osteoporosis doesn't show any signs in its early stages. Loss of bone density happens gradually, and people may not feel pain or discomfort.

2. Absence of Warning Indications

There are no warning indications of osteoporosis, such as discomfort, swelling, or redness. Lack of symptoms could cause people to be unaware of their illness.

3. Exploration Through Breaks:

Osteoporosis is frequently identified following a fracture, particularly one that affects the wrist, hip, or spine. Normal activity or mild trauma can cause these fractures.

4. Spinal Fractures:

In osteoporosis, vertebral (spine) fractures are prevalent. These fractures may result in kyphosis, a stooped look, or a loss of height. It's possible that these modifications won't be apparent right away.

5. Hip Breaks:

Osteoporosis-related hip fractures are a major problem that can have serious repercussions. They can raise morbidity and mortality rates and are frequently the consequence of a fall or other trauma.

6. Breaks to the Wrist:

A fall or collision can cause wrist fractures, especially in the distal radius. These fractures may be a sign of osteoporosis beneath the surface.

7. Dental Problems:

Jawbone problems, such as tooth loss or impaired dental health, can result from osteoporosis. These symptoms might not, however, be directly connected to a decrease in bone density.

8. Quiet Bone Loss:

Osteoporosis-related bone loss happens silently and painlessly. This quiet character emphasizes how crucial it is to take preventative steps, including bone density testing, to identify people who are at risk.

9. Assessing Bone Density:

One important osteoporosis diagnostic method is bone density testing, such as dual-energy X-ray absorptiometry (DXA) scans. These examinations assist in determining a person's risk of fracture and assessing bone mineral density.

10. Early intervention and prevention:

Osteoporosis is a quiet disease, thus early detection and prevention are essential. The condition can be managed and the risk of fractures decreased with the help of weight-bearing activity, appropriate nutrition, lifestyle changes, and prompt medical examination.

People need to take a proactive approach to maintaining their bone health, especially those who are more at risk. Frequent examinations, bone density tests, and consultations with medical experts can help with early identification and the application of preventative measures. Promoting bone health and avoiding problems related to bone fragility need knowledge of osteoporosis and its risk factors.

Testing for Bone Density

A crucial diagnostic technique for the evaluation and treatment of osteoporosis is bone density testing. These examinations, which are also known as bone mineral density (BMD) exams, offer numerical assessments of bone density at different body locations. Dual-energy X-ray absorptiometry is the most often utilized technique for determining bone density (DXA).

CHAPTER TWO

1. X-ray absorptiometry with dual energy (DXA):

The most popular and generally recognized technique for determining bone mineral density is DXA. It entails measuring bone density at particular locations, usually the hip and spine, using low-dose X-rays. A T-score, which contrasts a person's bone density with that of a healthy young adult of the same gender, is used to express the results.

2. Locations for Measurement:

Because osteoporotic fractures frequently occur at the hip and spine, DXA scans are frequently conducted there. Sometimes measurements are taken at other locations as well, such the forearm.

3. The Z- and T-scores:

The T-score measures a person's bone density in relation to a healthy young adult's peak bone density. A T-score of -1 or higher is regarded as normal; a value of -1 to -2.5 denotes osteoporosis; and a score of -2.5 or lower indicates low bone density (osteopenia). Bone density is compared to age-matched peers using the Z-score.

4. Evaluation of Fracture Risk:

A bone density test is useful in determining fracture risk, and those with low bone density are thought to be more susceptible to fractures. Healthcare providers use the findings as a basis when creating individualized management programs.

5. Keeping an eye on bone health

Testing for bone density on a regular basis is helpful in tracking changes in bone health over time. It aids in determining how well treatments and treatment plans maintain or increase bone density.

6. FRAX, the WHO Fracture Risk Assessment Tool:

Healthcare professionals may employ instruments like FRAX, which takes clinical risk factors into account to assess the 10-year probability of significant osteoporotic fractures, in addition to bone density tests. FRAX can assist in directing therapy choices.

7. Suggestions for Examination:

For postmenopausal women and men 50 years of age and above who have osteoporosis risk factors, bone density testing is advised. In younger people with certain risk factors, it might also be taken into consideration.

8. Testing Frequency:

The frequency of bone density testing is determined by the results and individual risk factors. Generally speaking, testing may be done less frequently for people at reduced risk or again every 1-2 years for those at higher risk.

Osteoporosis diagnosis, treatment, and early detection are greatly aided by bone density testing. It gives medical personnel useful information to evaluate fracture risk, direct therapies, and track the condition of bones over time. People who are at risk for osteoporosis should talk to their healthcare professionals about the best times and frequency to have bone density tests performed.

Methods of Therapy

Reducing the risk of fractures, increasing bone density, and slowing down bone loss are the goals of osteoporosis treatment. A combination of dietary therapies, lifestyle changes, and, occasionally, medication is used in treatment plans. The following are essential elements of osteoporosis treatment approaches:

1. Changes in Lifestyle:

Weight-Bearing Exercise: To strengthen and increase bone density, perform weight-bearing exercises including walking, running, and resistance training.

Balance and Strength Training: Include exercises that improve muscular strength and balance to lower the risk of fractures and falls.

Stop Smoking: Since smoking is linked to a higher risk of bone loss, give up smoking. Quitting smoking has been shown to improve bone health in general.

2. Sufficient Nutrition:

Calcium Intake: Make sure you get enough calcium each day from your food or from supplements. Mineralization of bone requires calcium.

Vitamin D Supplementation: Make sure you get enough vitamin D from sunshine exposure and, if needed, supplements. The absorption of calcium depends on vitamin D.

3. Drugs:

Bisphosphonates: These drugs, which include ibandronate, risedronate, and alendronate, help to prevent fractures by slowing the loss of bone. They frequently serve as osteoporosis's first line of treatment.

Selective Estrogen Receptor Modulators (SERMs): Drugs such as raloxifene imitate the actions of estrogen in specific tissues and can be administered to women who have gone through menopause in order to lower their risk of fracture.

Denosumab is a monoclonal antibody that can be injected every six months to prevent bone resorption.

Abaloparatide and Teriparatide: These drugs, which are parathyroid hormone derivatives, can promote the growth of new bone. Usually, they are only worn by those who are particularly susceptible to fractures.

4. Treatment with Hormone Replacement (HRT):

Hormone replacement therapy containing progesterone and estrogen may be taken into consideration for postmenopausal women in order to preserve bone density. A comprehensive risk-benefit analysis should inform the decision to use HRT, which should be unique to each patient.

5. Techniques for Preventing Falls:

Take steps to prevent falls because they are a common cause of fractures. This could involve vision tests, balance exercises, and home adjustments.

6. Frequent Observation:

Frequent monitoring of fracture risk and bone density aid in evaluating treatment efficacy and directing necessary modifications.

7. All-inclusive Care:

For those with osteoporosis, a multidisciplinary approach involving medical specialists such as endocrinologists, physical therapists, and orthopedic specialists can offer comprehensive care.

8. Tailored Care Programs:

Individualized treatment plans are frequently developed taking into account variables like age, sex, general health, and the existence of additional medical conditions. Healthcare professionals take into account each person's unique requirements and preferences.

Osteoporosis patients should collaborate closely with their medical team to create a customized treatment plan. Scheduling routine follow-up appointments enables continuous evaluation, treatment plan modifications, and resolution of any issues or alterations in bone health. A key element of long-term care to promote general bone health and lower the risk of fractures is lifestyle adjustments and preventive measures.

Lifestyle Modifications for Strong Bones

Osteoporosis management and prevention depend heavily on maintaining bone health. Adopting certain lifestyle practices can help maintain bone density and lower the chance of fractures. The following are important lifestyle choices that can help maintain bone health in the setting of osteoporosis:

1. Sufficient Intake of Calcium:

Make sure you get enough calcium each day, as this is an essential mineral for strong bones. To help meet calcium needs, foods like dairy products, leafy greens, fortified foods, and calcium supplements, if needed, can be consumed.

2. Supplementing with Vitamin D:

Retain ideal levels of vitamin D by combining sun exposure with vitamin D supplements, if necessary. Vitamin D is necessary for healthy bones and helps the body absorb calcium.

3. A well-rounded diet

Eat a diet high in fruits, vegetables, whole grains, lean proteins, and balance to ensure optimal health. Essential nutrients for overall health, including bone health, can be found in a well-rounded diet.

4. Exercise Using Weights:

Take part in weight-bearing activities like resistance training, dancing, walking, and running. These exercises build stronger bones, increase bone density, and improve general strength.

5. Strength and Resistance Exercises:

Incorporate strength training exercises into your routine to maintain and grow muscular mass. Sturdy muscles help to maintain total stability by supporting the bones.

6. Fall Safety Procedures:

Put fall prevention measures into practice because falls can result in fractures. This include utilizing handrails, keeping your home clutter-free, and taking care of any possible hazards.

7. Quitting Smoking:

Give up smoking since it increases the risk of fractures and increased bone loss. Quitting smoking improves cardiovascular and bone health in general.

8. Restrict Your Alcohol Use:

Limit alcohol consumption because it can have a detrimental effect on bone health. To preserve bone density, moderation is essential.

9. Keep Your Weight in Check:

Sustain a healthy body weight by combining appropriate diet with frequent exercise. Bone loss may be exacerbated by extreme weight reduction or underweight conditions.

10. Body mechanics and posture: - Maintain optimal body mechanics and posture to lower your risk of fractures, particularly those to the spine. Steer clear of activities that require a lot of twisting and bending.

11. Regular Medical Examinations: Make an appointment for routine examinations with

medical professionals to evaluate bone health and talk about any changes in risk factors or concerns.

12. Limit Caffeine Intake: - Restrict your caffeine intake to avoid overindulging, as this may cause problems with calcium absorption. Moderation is recommended, particularly for those who are at risk of osteoporosis.

13. Be Aware of drugs: - Recognize which drugs, such as some corticosteroids and anticonvulsants, may have an adverse effect on bone health. Consult with healthcare professionals about any possible hazards, and when needed, look into other solutions.

14. Maintain Hydration: Water is vital for good health, which includes strong bones. Make sure you are drinking plenty of it.

15. Adequate Sleep: Getting enough good sleep is important for general health, which includes bone health.

Using these lifestyle changes in conjunction with a comprehensive approach to bone health can help manage and prevent osteoporosis. It's crucial to speak with healthcare professionals to receive tailored guidance based on unique requirements and risk factors. Whole health and long-term bone health are enhanced by routine check-ups and lifestyle modifications.

CHAPTER THREE

Safety precautions and fall prevention

For those who have osteoporosis, preventing falls is essential since they can result in fractures and other problems. There is a significant reduction in the risk of falls with the use of safety measures and lifestyle modifications. For those with osteoporosis, the following safety and fall prevention measures are recommended:

1. Improvements to the Home:

Get rid of anything that can trip people up, like cords, rugs, and clutter near walkways.

To stop people from slipping, place non-slip mats in the kitchen and restroom.

Install grab bars in the restroom, paying particular attention to the areas beside the shower and toilet.

Make sure your home is well-lit throughout, and use nightlights in the restrooms and corridors.

2. Footwear

Put on supportive, robust shoes with non-slip soles.

Steer clear of smooth-soled shoes or socks when navigating slick surfaces.

3. Assisting Instruments:

If you need assistance staying upright, use walkers or canes.

When engaging in outdoor activities, think about using a walking stick or trekking poles.

4. Consistent Exercise:

Try some strength and balance-building workouts like yoga or tai chi.

Adhere to a customized fitness regimen intended to improve your general stability.

5. Review of Medication:

Review drug interactions and side effects with medical professionals on a regular basis to determine how they might impact balance or coordination.

6. Eye Exam:

To maintain good eyesight and quickly treat any visual problems, have frequent eye exams.

7. Evaluation of Bone Density:

Test your bone density frequently to keep an eye on your bone health and determine your risk of fracture.

8. Sufficient Vitamin D and Calcium:

To maintain bone health, make sure you're getting enough calcium and vitamin D.

To find out if supplements are required, speak with your healthcare providers.

9. Programs for Fall Prevention:

Take advantage of community-based fall prevention programs or balance training courses.

10. Remain Mobile and Active: Steer clear of extended periods of idleness. Strength and flexibility are maintained with regular movement.

11. fluids: Maintain adequate fluids because dehydration can impair coordination and balance.

12. Regular Medical Examinations: Make an appointment with your doctor on a regular basis to discuss any health concerns that might affect your ability to move around or balance.

13. Recognize Environmental Hazards: - Exercise caution when negotiating stairs, uneven terrain, and dimly lit areas.

When climbing or descending steps, use the handrails.

14. Use Hip Protectors: - Take into consideration using hip protectors, particularly if there has been a history of fractures or falls.

15. Become Acquainted with Emergency Protocols: - Recognize emergency protocols and prepare a strategy in the event of an accident or fall.

16. Maintain a Healthy Lifestyle: - Make healthy lifestyle choices, such as eating a balanced diet, getting regular exercise, and abstaining from tobacco and alcohol usage.

Fall prevention is a cooperative endeavor including patients and medical professionals.

People with osteoporosis can lower their chance of fractures and falls by adopting these safety precautions into their daily lives, improving their general safety and wellbeing. An efficient fall prevention plan includes proactive management of osteoporosis and regular communication with healthcare practitioners.

Managing Osteoporosis

Managing the difficulties brought on by osteoporosis requires a blend of practical, psychological, and physical coping mechanisms. The following are coping mechanisms for those who have osteoporosis:

1. Understanding and knowledge:

Find more about the causes, symptoms, and treatment options for osteoporosis. Being aware of the illness enables people to take an active role in their own care.

2. Interaction with Medical Professionals:

Keep lines of communication open and consistent with medical professionals. Talk about any worries, signs, or modifications to your bone health.

3. Assistance System:

Create a solid support system with your loved ones, friends, and medical professionals. Discuss your worries and experiences with people who can empathize and offer emotional support.

4. Working Out:

Regularly perform low-impact workouts to keep your muscles strong and flexible. Create a personalized fitness program in collaboration with a physical therapist.

5. Dietary Guidelines and Supplements:

Adopt a healthy, calcium- and vitamin-D-rich diet. Consult your healthcare physician about the need for supplements.

6. Avoiding Falls:

Reduce the risk of fractures by putting fall prevention techniques into practice. This covers making adjustments to your home, utilizing assistive technology, and taking part in fall prevention initiatives.

7. Adherence to Medication:

Follow the recommended course of treatment and medication. Address any worries or adverse reactions with medical professionals.

8. Psychological Wellness:

Talk about the psychological effects of osteoporosis. If necessary, seek assistance from mental health specialists.

9. Technology that adapts:

If required, use assistive technology like braces, walkers, or canes. These gadgets can improve freedom and movement.

10. Pain Management: Under the supervision of medical professionals, experiment with pain management strategies like heat or cold therapy, relaxation techniques, and over-the-counter pain medicines.

11. Lifestyle Modifications: - To reduce joint stress, modify your lifestyle to include good body mechanics. Steer clear of activities that could put you at risk for fractures.

12. Regular Exams: Make an appointment for routine examinations with medical professionals to monitor bone health, evaluate the efficacy of treatment, and make any required modifications.

13. Attend Support Groups: - Take into consideration attending osteoporosis support groups, where you can meet people going through comparable struggles, exchange stories, and learn coping mechanisms from one another.

14. Emphasize Independence: In your day-to-day activities, emphasize your independence. Determine the tactics and assistive technology that improve autonomy.

15. Holistic Approach: - Take a comprehensive approach to health, taking into account social and emotional factors in addition to physical ones. Take part in things that make you happy and fulfilled.

16. Plan for the Future: - Make the required preparations to keep a supportive living environment in place and think about long-term care choices.

17. Keep Up to Date: - Remain updated on developments in the study and management of osteoporosis. Having knowledge enables people to make well-informed decisions regarding their health.

18. Retain an optimistic outlook: Encourage an optimistic outlook. Rather than concentrating on what cannot be done to improve well-being, consider what can be done.

Osteoporosis management is a dynamic process that calls for constant self-management, medical specialists' assistance, and an optimistic outlook. Despite the difficulties presented by osteoporosis, people can improve their quality of life and keep their independence by actively treating both the physical and emotional components of the condition. Effective coping and long-term well-being are facilitated by proactive measures, open communication, and routine examinations.

CONCLUSION

In summary, osteoporosis is a chronic disorder marked by bone weakening that increases fragility and raises the risk of fractures. Even while osteoporosis is frequently asymptomatic in its early stages, its effects become apparent when fractures happen, especially in weight-bearing bones like the wrists, hips, and spine.

A multimodal strategy is important for the effective care of osteoporosis, and it incorporates fall prevention techniques, weight-bearing exercise, appropriate diet, lifestyle adjustments, and, when necessary, medicines. In order to effectively treat the illness over time, regular monitoring with bone density tests and open contact with healthcare specialists are essential.

Creating a support system, learning about osteoporosis, and having an optimistic outlook all help a person deal with the difficulties that come with having the disease. Giving people the information and resources they need to take care of themselves improves their capacity to live active, satisfying lives in spite of the effects of osteoporosis.

For those with osteoporosis, there is hope for better results and a higher quality of life due to ongoing research, therapeutic advancements, and a holistic approach to bone health. Individuals can keep their independence and general well-being by navigating the path with resilience by addressing both the physical and emotional aspects of the condition. A proactive mindset, preventive measures, and routine examinations are the cornerstones of an effective long-term osteoporosis care strategy.

THE END